MALE SURVIVAL GUIDE

for
PREGNANCY,
DELIVERY,
and the
POST PARTUM PERIOD

John T. Scully, M.D.
Kimberly Ann Scully, R.N.

Canada • UK • Ireland • USA • Spain

Note for Librarians: a cataloguing record for this book that includes Dewey Decimal
Classification and US Library of Congress numbers is available from the Library and
Archives of Canada. The complete cataloguing record can be obtained from their
online database at:
www.collectionscanada.ca/amicus/index-e.html
ISBN 1-4120-3644-5
Printed in Victoria, BC, Canada

TRAFFORD

Offices in Canada, USA, Ireland, UK and Spain
This book was published *on-demand* in cooperation with Trafford Publishing. On-
demand publishing is a unique process and service of making a book available for
retail sale to the public taking advantage of on-demand manufacturing and Internet
marketing. On-demand publishing includes promotions, retail sales, manufacturing,
order fulfilment, accounting and collecting royalties on behalf of the author.
Book sales in Europe:
Trafford Publishing (UK) Ltd., Enterprise House, Wistaston Road Business Centre,
Wistaston Road, Crewe CW2 7RP UNITED KINGDOM
phone 01270 251 396 (local rate 0845 230 9601)
facsimile 01270 254 983; orders.uk@trafford.com
Book sales for North America and international:
Trafford Publishing, 6E–2333 Government St.,
Victoria, BC V8T 4P4 CANADA
phone 250 383 6864 (toll-free 1 888 232 4444)
fax 250 383 6804; email to orders@trafford.com
Order online at:
www.trafford.com/robots/04-1472.html

10 9 8 7 6 5 4 3 2

Dedication

We would like to dedicate this document to the near 20,000 Mothers and Fathers who allowed us to take part in the making of their families. Thank you for the trust.

We would also like to salute the wonderful Nurses at St. Peter's University Hospital who assisted us in this undertaking. We could never have done it without them.

The woman about to become a mother, or with her new-born infant upon her bosom should be the object of trembling care and sympathy wherever she bears her tender burden, or stretches her aching limbs. The very outcast of the street has pity upon her sister in degradation when the seal of promised maternity is impressed upon her. The remorseless vengeance of the law, brought down upon its victim by a machinery as sure as destiny, is arrested in its fall at a word, which reveals her transient claim for mercy. The solemn prayer of the liturgy singles out her sorrows from the multiple trials of life, to plead for her in the hour of peril. God forbid that any member of the profession to which she trusts her life, doubly precious at that eventful period, should hazard it negligently, unadvisedly, or selfishly!

William Jennings Bryant

Table of Contents

Introduction

I do not think that I shall ever forget the joy and wonder that I felt when I first attended a woman giving birth. It happened some forty or so years ago at a small maternity clinic in a very poor section of Mexico City. The equipment was modest and the surroundings humble, but the birth of a child is a miracle no matter where it occurs, be it a palace or a hut. To see this blue, almost lifeless infant come into the world and let out its first cry of protest was beyond description. Now, some nine, or so, thousand deliveries later, the thrill is still there. Maybe the original awe has been somewhat dampened but, not that feeling of being present at something grand and wonderful. Little of that had changed.

But, **having** a baby has changed over the past forty years. One of the greatest changes has been the participation of the father in the birth process. In the past, his biggest role was to boil the proverbial water. I can remember when we treated the expectant father as if he were a leper. The closest he was able to get to Labor and Delivery was to drop off his wife at the entrance door. There they were left either to sit in a room the size of a linen closet or to go out for "a few beers". This was their **Confinement!!!** Little information concerning their wife's progress was given until the doctor came out to announce the sex of the baby.

Little by little, much like a slow moving flow of hot lava, the fathers began to gain entrance to the "Holy of Holies" — The Labor Room. It was here, much like a lump on a log, they were permitted to watch their wife labor. Yet they were still excluded from the birth of their child. For once it was time to go to the delivery room they were again sent off to the Father's Waiting Room.

The lava kept flowing. A great demand arose to allow them to be present at the birth of their child. Such audacity! One man even handcuffed himself to his wife in order to guarantee his presence. He almost spent the night in jail.

All of which brings us to where we are today. **FULL PARTICIPATION** by the father in the birth of his child from the beginning till the end. Gentlemen, whether you like it or not, you are expected to participate. Just as it was taken for granted some forty years ago that you would not participate but wait in the waiting room; it is now expected that you will participate. How lucky you are. Therefore, I do hope that this book will help you in this undertaking. Believe me, it is a beautiful event that you shouldn't miss. I promise you that you will never forget it. What a gift!

PART ONE

PREGNANCY

Chapter One

HOW DID IT HAPPEN?

Forgive me if I assume that your mate is now or soon to be pregnant. If not, you have little need for this book. If my assumption is correct, the first question that needs to be answered is "How did it happen?"

This question is not meant to insult your intelligence. I am sure you know how it happened... sexual intercourse. What I would like you to understand is the mechanism of conception.

Each month a woman's body prepares itself for pregnancy. It is called the menstrual cycle. The *Preparation for Pregnancy Cycle* really would be a more appropriate designation since this is what it's all about. The menstrual period has been referred to as the "uterine shedding its tears of frustration".

It all starts in the pituitary gland in the brain, which makes a hormone that stimulates the lining of the uterus to grow. This could be compared to a gardener putting down topsoil. Approximately fourteen days from the last menstrual period an egg explodes from the ovary into the abdominal cavity. This leaves behind a small cyst which makes a second hormone, progesterone. Progesterone, in turn, enriches the lining of the uterus to make it more of a well-nourished layer for the implantation of the fertilized egg. You could compare this to the farmer adding fertilizer to the topsoil before planting his seed. Within seven to ten days the lining of the uterus is ready to accept the fertilized egg for implantation. If there is no fertilized egg, this lining is cast off (menstruation) and the process begins again.

If you go back to the magical day 14 when the egg explodes from the ovary, we can follow its progress to conception or death. The egg is picked up by the end of the fallopian tube much like a vacuum cleaner would pick up dust. The fallopian tube is, as it is called, a tube that is connected at one end to the inside of the uterus and is opened at the other end and lies near the ovary. The egg, unlike the sperm, has no means of self-propulsion. The fallopian tube has millions of microscopic hairlike cells that line the inside of the tube. It is with these cells that wave back and forth, that the egg is moved along the tube to its final destination, the inside of the uterus. If the sperm, deposited in the vagina during intercourse, can live through the arduous journey up the mouth of the uterus, past the inside of the uterus and into the fallopian tube, conception may occur. But, the sperm must meet the egg at the proper time and place for this to occur. If the sperm arrives after the egg has been out of the ovary for over twelve hours, the egg will be most likely dead and not able to be fertilized. If the sperm arrives too soon, all is not lost, since they can live for days inside the female awaiting the arrival of the egg. If fertilized, the egg, with twenty three chromosomes and the sperm with its twenty three chromosomes combine, we have a forty six chromosomes cell that will then divide into two cells, then four cells, then eight cells as it makes its way down the tube to the uterus. The lining of the uterus, now prepared, awaits the arrival of the fertilized egg for implantation. We now have the beginning of a new life.

Chapter Two

NINE MONTHS DO NOT A PREGNANCY MAKE

Ask anyone anywhere, be they an Ivy League graduate or the most humble of the poor and they all will tell you that it takes nine months from the beginning to the end to give birth to a baby. T'aint so! The average pregnancy last 280 days or 40 weeks from the last menstrual period. What makes it so confusing is that most people add nine months to the last period to calculate the due date. Nine months are 39 weeks. They inadvertently shorten the time by one week. As an example, if the last menstrual period was January 1st, the due date, by their reckoning, would be October 1st or nine months (39 weeks) later. The due date by the 40 week rule would be October 7th. I know that this sounds insignificant to you but, believe me to a pregnant woman that extra week seems like a month not seven days.

Now, add to this confusion that anything between two weeks before the due date and two weeks after the due date is considered a normal length or pregnancy. Or the fact that a twin pregnancy is usually, on average, three weeks shorter than a singleton. The same can be said for triplets, which come earlier than a twin pregnancy. And so forth. The more babies, the shorter the pregnancy.

This makes for a great deal of stress for the whole family, but mainly for the mother who is bombarded with phone calls asking her, "didn't you deliver yet?" That is why the due date is called the expected date of confinement. It's just that … expected. It's a ballpark figure. It is not written in stone. If the due date is June 2nd and your wife wakes up on the morning of the third still pregnant, be cool. It's not a crisis.

Chapter Three

THE FIRST TRIMESTER

She thinks she looks good but feels terrible.

Pregnancies are divided, for the sake of description, into trimesters; three-month segments of thirteen plus weeks each. Each trimester has its own trials and tribulations. The first trimester, starting at the last period, is one of great physical and psychological changes.

As the uterus grows from the size of a lemon, when not pregnant, to the size of a small grapefruit at 13 plus weeks it exerts pressure on the urinary bladder. This pressure causes the bladder to reduce its capacity to hold the usual amount of urine and in turn causes the pregnant lady to need to empty her bladder much more frequently. It is not necessarily painful but it can be very annoying.

The same is true of the rectum. It too is affected by the enlarging uterus and some women have trouble with constipation at this stage of pregnancy.

Another common change in early pregnancy is growth of the breasts. Some women of small size find this a plus while others can be very distressed at the enlargement. Husbands take note. Never, I mean, never, say that you would love it if the growth could last forever. Remember you loved her for the woman that she is, not the one you wish she were.

The first trimester is the time of miscarriages. Usually, these occur around week 8-10. The majority of these are chromosomally defective fetuses. The old Hollywood dramatics where a woman loses a pregnancy after a fall is nonsense. It takes more than a fall to end a healthy pregnancy. In reality, there is little that can be done to avoid a miscarriage. If the pregnancy is doomed, it's doomed.

Morning sickness is sometimes present during the first trimester. It can range from a little nausea now and then that is made better with frequent small meals to an outright dangerous situation that requires hospitalization. Any protracted vomiting should be reported to the doctor. The lack of caloric intake at this stage of pregnancy is of little importance, but the lack of liquids can be very dangerous. Dehydration is very dangerous to both the mother and the fetus. No matter how much she may be vomiting, try to help her to take fluids until you have contacted the doctor.

It is very important that the first visit to the doctor be made during the first trimester. It is during these early weeks that a diagnosis of a pregnancy can be made and the assurance that the pregnancy is in the right place. Pregnancies outside the uterus (ectopic pregnancies) can be very dangerous and the earlier they are diagnosed the better. We will discuss this further in another chapter.

It is also during the first trimester that many important blood tests need to be done. A blood count is done to make sure that Mom is not anemic. An anemic person has a decreased ability to carry oxygen to the organs within her body, but what is very important is that she also has a decreased capacity to carry oxygen to the baby. She will need to have this corrected as it is also important later in pregnancy when bleeding can be a problem and if she starts off already compromised she can get behind the proverbial "eight ball".

It is also important to know her blood type and her Rh factor, as there are situations when the mother's blood types or Rh factors can be in conflict with the baby's. It is also important to know if the mother has any antibodies in her blood that may cause problems. This will be discussed more thoroughly later.

It is also important to know if the mother is immune to German measles. For, a mother who is still susceptible to German measles and contracted the disease in the first trimester she now has a big problem with the disease that can cause severe problems in the baby. As an aside, every woman should know her German measles status **before** she gets pregnant, not after. If she knows that she is susceptible she can be given an injection to make her immune.

It is also important to know whether or not she has ever had Chicken Pox. An outbreak of Chicken Pox in early pregnancy can also be harmful to the baby.

It is also important to know if the mother has ever had Hepatitis. If so, the baby's doctor will give the baby an injection at birth to protect him/her.

The same is true for HIV. The mother can be treated to protect her baby should she unfortunately be positive for HIV.

An up to date Pap smear is in order. Just because a woman is pregnant it does not mean that she is protected from infections or abnormal Pap Smears.

As you can see, it is better to lock the barn door before the horse runs away. There are many things that can be either corrected or at least treated if found out early. There are things, if found out later in pregnancy, which can have already done their harm.

I would highly recommend that those planning a pregnancy go through a pre-pregnancy session with their doctor. Anyone with a family history of Cystic Fibrosis needs screening. Jewish couples should know their Tay Sacks status. The list is long but the studies are worth the effort.

A word about miscarriage: Miscarriages usually occur around 8-10 weeks into the pregnancy. They begin with vaginal bleeding somewhat heavier than a menstrual period and can be accompanied by cramps and the passage of clots. The bleeding is not as alarming as a miscarriage near the end of the first trimester. This can be quite heavy. Losses in the second trimester can be profuse. It is best to report any bleeding to the doctor, no matter when it occurs in a pregnancy.

An ultrasound exam done during the first trimester is of great help. It can rectify the real age of the pregnancy in those patients whose dates of their last menstrual period are not known. It also can detect the presence of a multiple pregnancy at an early stage, which is of great help in managing the pregnancy. Prior to the use of ultrasound up to fifty percent of all multiple pregnancies were not know until delivery.

There is also another condition called hydatidiform mole. This is a condition in which the after birth undergoes a cystic degeneration and destroys the pregnancy. It needs to be removed for it does have the potential to become a malignancy. Years ago this was uniformly fatal. Today, it is highly curable if found early. Ultrasound can pick this up very early.

It is very important that the expectant mothers not smoke, consume alcohol or use drugs as these can be dangerous to the baby. It is a great time for both the mother and the father to stop smoking. If Mom smokes so, does the baby. If Dad smokes, Mom can still inhale his smoke and in turn affect the baby. Considering the health hazards of drugs and nicotine and the high cost of cigarettes, if the money spent on these bad habits was put in the bank for the baby, by the time he/she wanted to go to college you would have enough money to pay for it.

It would be good for you to be informed of the Bastion of Medical knowledge, The Hair Dressers. More erroneous information is passed between pregnant and non-pregnant women while at the hairdressers than probably at any other place. Everyone is an expert and they have their ghost stories to tell. All negative. It's like the world. Bad news is always circulated and good news is not. Help your wife to resist this onslaught of scary stories by telling her to check it all out with the doctor. Most "Old Wives' tales" are nonsense.

Chapter Four

THE SECOND TRIMESTER

Looks good/Feels good.

From the mother's point of view, the second trimester is probably the best part of the pregnancy. She is past the nausea stage. The breasts have stabilized and she feels more comfortable with them. The uterus has grown out of the pelvis and is now up and into the spaciousness of the abdominal cavity. She is no longer bothered with urinary frequency. She hasn't yet gotten to the stage where she is so big that she is uncomfortable with her massive belly. In a word, she feels great. She even glows with the self-satisfaction of pending motherhood. Take this opportunity to tell her how great she looks and how much you love her for in the next trimester she is going to be filled with many doubts and she needs you to support her. A surprise gift would be nice. A weekend away would help. Remember that in a short time you are going to have a baby that needs your full attention and it will be hard to get away for a while. It will do you both good.

The baby starts the second trimester fully formed with all the necessary parts, but small. He/she will spend the next 13 weeks growing from the size of a few ounces to about a pound. This is not the rapid growth of the last trimester but a very important stage in its development. Should the baby be delivered during this trimester the chance of survival is nil. Perhaps at the very end of the second trimester, say 25-26 weeks, there is a chance but it's not the best. It is best to get the pregnancy into the last (third) trimester where the baby gains about a half a pound a week. If it gained that much in the second trimester it would weigh about six pounds at 26 weeks, which it does not.

One of the major problems in the second trimester is an incompetent cervix. This is when, for reasons not fully known, the mouth of the womb (uterus) instead of staying long and closed until labor progressively opens up and the fetus is expelled. If caught in time, this can be treated with good results, by sewing closed the mouth of the womb. Catching it in time is the problem. Having a woman who has lost a baby at this stage in a previous pregnancy should be a warning sign and the mouth of the womb can be examined on a frequent basis. This is done visually and by ultrasound examination. Women who have had surgery on their cervix should be suspect. Some symptoms include a watery discharge or staining or a feeling of vaginal fullness. Unfortunately, most first time losses go undiagnosed due to a lack of any alerting signs or symptoms.

Another cause of a mid pregnancy loss is a condition where the small blood vessels that feed the placenta become clogged and thereby restrict the blood flow to that very important part of the pregnancy and thereby cause the loss of the pregnancy. This too, like the incompetent cervix, is seldom diagnosed the first time. The diagnosis is usually made after repeated mid pregnancy losses. Certain blood tests are then done and if they indicate this condition the woman is treated in the next pregnancy. The treatments vary from baby aspirin, to prednisone, to heparin, all in the attempt to eradicate the formation of the micro clots in the small vessels feeding the placenta.

Testing that is usually done in the second trimester: Quad Screen. To understand this you need to understand Down's Syndrome. Down's syndrome (see that section) is statistically more common in women 35 and older. This does not mean that younger women cannot have a Down's baby. They can, but the probability of a loss of the pregnancy if an amniocentesis is done in a younger woman out weighs the probability of a Down's baby. Therefore it is not advised to routinely do amniocentesis on younger women for more babies will be lost to miscarriage than the finding of

Down's babies. With this in mind, a group of blood tests were developed to test whether or not a younger woman was acting her age, so to speak or was she acting as if she were 35 or older. This then could be used to advise women of their risk of, Down's syndrome. The woman could then make a decision whether or not she wished to have an amniocentesis performed. Also, one of tests, Alpha fetoprotein, is a particular marker for neural tube defects (Spina bifida, etc.) in the fetus. This is usually followed up with a targeted ultrasound to examine the baby's nervous system.

In the hands of a well-trained Sonographer and a Perinatologist an ultrasound directed at various parts of the fetal anatomy can have a very high success in diagnosing Down's Syndrome. It is not as efficient as an amniocentesis but it has no risk of fetal loss, which makes it somewhat more acceptable to some mothers. This test is usually done at 18 weeks and the results are known immediately. The genetic amniocentesis is usually done at 16 weeks and the results can take about 2-3 weeks.

There is also a test for genetic information called a chorionic villus biopsy. This is done by passing a small tube up through the mouth of the womb and taking a biopsy of fetal tissue. It is done under ultrasound guidance. Its advantages are that it is done around 12 weeks of pregnancy and the results take about 2-3 weeks. The disadvantages are that it is not uniformly available in that it takes a great deal of practice to become adept at it. Also, there is some evidence that there is an increase of injury to the limbs of the fetus.

At twenty weeks usually an ultrasound is done to verify the normalcy of the fetus. It is also at this time that the sex of the fetus can be determined. Some parents are anxious to know this, while others are not. It's all up to you. If you want to know, ask. If you don't what to know tell the sonographer and look the other way when you are told to. Sometimes, if no ultrasound was done earlier in the pregnancy, we learn of the presence of more than one baby. This is not only nice for the parents to know, but very important to the physician. The care of a multiple pregnancy is very different from that of a singleton. More about this in "Multiple Pregnancies".

Chapter Five

THE THIRD TRIMESTER

Looks bad/Feels bad.

This is a very good time to listen to Neil Diamond and B. Streisand's "You don't bring me flowers." And bring her flowers and tell her you love her.

The third trimester is one of growth. A normal baby will gain about a half pound a week during these last 13 weeks. And it is this end to which your doctor will strive to avoid prematurity and certain problems that are found during this time.

From the mother's point of view this is a period of progressive discomfort. Each week her belly is getting bigger. Near the end she probably will have trouble just tying her shoes. In fact now she probably will wear slip on footwear exclusively. She no longer feels attractive. Dad here is your chance to be a prince. Don't miss an opportunity to tell her she looks great and you love her. Remember she's carrying your child inside her. Something you can't do and probably wouldn't do if you could. Surprise her with an appointment to have a manicure and a pedicure. She'll never forget your kindness and she needs a great deal of love and appreciation right now. Also, keep in mind that down the road she is going into the scary land of childbirth. Much as we try, no one can predict what it will be like and her head is filled with all the erroneous facts that she was given by her well-meaning friends at the hairdressers. I guarantee you that much of what she had heard is wrong and what's worse it is negative. Most people prefer to spread bad news and keep the good to themselves.

Some women become unable to handle sugar in the later part of pregnancy. They become what is called a gestational diabetic. It is for this that she is tested at about 28 weeks to see how she handles a sugar load. She is given a drink high in sugar and her blood sugar level is checked. If it is high it then needs to be determined if this can be controlled with a diet low in sugar or if it is necessary for her to be put on insulin therapy. In either event, it changes the course of the remainder of the pregnancy. But if handled correctly it should create no problem. The problems arise when the tests are not done and the diagnosis is not made or when Mom doesn't follow the direction of the doctor.

Another test done at 28 weeks is to check if an Rh negative mother is developing any antibodies against Rh positive blood. This needs an explanation. If the mother is Rh negative it really means that her blood does not contain the Rh factor. This means nothing in and of itself. It gains importance in pregnancy. If the Rh negative mother is carrying an Rh positive baby their bloods are incompatible. If any of the baby's Rh positive blood gets into the mother's blood stream her defense mechanisms make antibodies to neutralize the Rh factor that is foreign to her. She, in a word, destroys the red blood cells of the baby that made their way into her body. At this stage, all is well for her and for the baby. But, should she make enough antibodies and they pass back to the baby the antibodies will destroy the baby's Rh positive red blood cells. This can be anything from a slight anemia in the baby to a grave danger to his/hers well being. Therefore, if the test shows that she has made anti Rh antibodies she must be followed very closely to determine how extensive this production is. The baby too must be followed very closely so as to deliver him/her when it is mature but before it is severely affected by blood destruction. If the mother is not making antibodies she is given an injection (Rhogam) to curb her from making antibodies for the next 12 weeks. Once the baby is born its blood is typed. If it is Rh negative nothing further is done for their bloods are compatible. If it is Rh positive the baby is tested to see if it has been subjected to Rh positive antibodies. If it has then the baby needs to be worked up to see how severe this may be. If it turns out that the baby is Rh positive and is fine and a new antibody test on the mother fails to show antibodies, she is given another injection of Rhogam to combat any Rh positive fetal blood test that may have passed into her blood during the delivery.

There is a group of problems in the last trimester that I will group as Toxemias. They come with many different names such as pre eclampsia, eclampsia, pregnancy induced hypertension. H.E.E.L.P. syndrome, etc. This would be a book in itself. I will try to give you a general overview of these very complicated situations. Generally speaking these situations are of unknown cause and present themselves with various levels of excess weight gain, water retention, increase blood pressure and presence of proteins in the urine. The definitive treatment is delivery. But, depending on the stage of pregnancy at which they present themselves and the degree of severity of the symptoms it can be like being between a rock and a hard place. The mother is at great risk and if born the baby is at a stage of pregnancy when survival is dubious.

The treatment, if there is only mild blood pressure elevation, is bed rest. Anything more severe than that requires hospitalization. Attempts will be made to prolong the pregnancy and lower the blood pressure. At times these two aims are at odds with each other and decisions are very hard on everyone. If time permits, the mother will be given steroids to accelerate the maturity of the infant's lungs so that should it be a premature delivery some aid will have been given to the baby.

Prematurity is a consideration of the last trimester. Up to approximately 35 weeks any labor is considered premature labor and it is treated in two ways. One, the mother is given steroid to protect the baby's lungs should he/she deliver. The other is to give the mother one of the drugs that are used to attempt to stop the labor. Sometimes it works and sometimes it doesn't. When it works everybody is happy. When it doesn't, it's up to the Neonatologist to care for the premature infant.

Premature rupture of the membranes. Aside from rupture of the membranes within the last few weeks of pregnancy, rupture of membranes can be very troublesome. Much depends on when it happens. Should it happen at, say 20 weeks, the baby cannot survive if born at this time. Likewise, if the baby or the mother becomes infected the problems are compounded. The baby is in danger and so is the mother. Attempts to prolong the pregnancy can lead to severe maternal complication, including the loss of the uterus due to infection or even loss of the mother. The baby is a lost cause. He/she will not last long in a uterus that is infected and will die. If the mother does not become infected and the mere rupturing of the membranes in itself does not start premature labor the problems are not over. There is the worry that should the amount of fluid needed for the baby not be reformed, the baby could suffer great deformities or even a loss of the formation of its lung (Aplastic Lungs). This too could lead to the death of the baby soon after birth.

Yet, it is possible to rupture membranes at say 20 weeks and suffer no bad effects. It is only necessary for labor not to start and for no infection to take over and lastly for the baby to produce enough fluid for its environment.

Placental Problems. Most of the problems of the placenta have to do with its location or with its depth of implantation.

First location: The placenta can be located anywhere within the uterus as long as it is not near or covering the mouth of the womb. If it is so located it is called Placenta Previa. If a small portion of it is near the edge of the opening, it is called a marginal Placenta Previa. If it is covering a part of the opening, it is called a partial Placenta Previa. If it covers the whole opening, it is called a Total Placenta Previa. A low lying placenta is near the mouth of the womb but is not a placenta previa and gives little if any problems. Placenta previas that are diagnosed in the first trimester can migrate up and out of harms way as the pregnancy progresses. Those that are diagnosed later do not.

The usual first symptom is painless vaginal bleeding around the end of the first trimester and the beginning of the third (26 plus weeks). It can be anywhere from light bleeding to profuse bleeding. This happens because at this stage of pregnancy the lower part of the uterus, around the mouth, begins to pull up and shorten. This can cause a shearing off of the placenta. The amount of bleeding is related to the amount of shearing. It can be self-limiting but usually it will recur and be more dangerous with each new episode of bleeding. The trick is to prolong the pregnancy as much as possible and control the mother's health with blood transfusions. How to deliver the baby is another problem. It goes without saying that a total placenta previa will require a cesarean section, for the placenta is a total barrier to delivery through the mouth of the womb. The less the opening is covered the more likely that a vaginal birth is possible. But, should the bleeding be too profuse, a cesarean section will be done no matter the extent of the coverage.

Depth of implantation of the placenta: The placenta should be implanted deep enough to pick up nourishments from the mother but not so deep that it can not be detached after the birth of the baby. These are called placenta accretas. If the depth is so deep that it involves the muscular part of the womb these are called placenta incretas. And if they are through the full thickness of the uterus and may even invade adjacent organs, as the bladder, they are called placenta percretas. These invasions not only vary in their depth but also vary in the amount of the placenta that is so involved. In any event they can be very dangerous and frequently require a hysterectomy.

Chapter Six

WHAT IS IT LIKE TO BECOME A MOTHER?

I'd like to take you through a pregnancy from a woman's point of view. I really don't think that most men have any idea of what it is like, so here goes.

Once a woman realizes she is pregnant she frequently is bothered with "morning sickness". A misnomer if there ever was one. It is nausea, and at times vomiting, at any time of day not just the morning. It can be a small annoyance or so severe that hospitalization is required. Food that she likes is now awful and food that she was not that fond of she craves. The mere smell of food can trigger an attack. You may want to go out to dinner and she can barely get out of the bathroom. This can continue through the first 12-13 weeks of pregnancy. She looks and feels terrible. It's not in her head. It's real. Be considerate of this and help her out. If she wants pigs' knuckles, get them for her. Forget the foods that your mother told you she should eat during pregnancy. She will have ample time to catch up once the nausea goes away.

What's next? The breasts enlarge and can be uncomfortable or even painful. The discomfort will pass, but this is not the time for you to admire her voluptuousness. She really prefers that you love the original. That's the woman you are going to spend the rest of your life with. She is also the mother of your child.

As the weeks progress she is going to become bigger in girth. Think of yourself developing a big beer belly in six months; if you don't already have one. It gets to the point that she can't tie her shoelaces and she begins to wear shoes that do not need to be tied. Of course, she may not be able to see her feet for that matter. Each time she goes to the doctor the nurse is going to give her a cup a littler bigger than a shot glass. She is expected to be able to see well enough to urinate into this small receptacle. You, of course, would have no trouble doing this for you have a pointer (penis). Even though, beer belly or not, you frequently miss the bowl.

As she gets bigger there is a chance she will develop "stretch marks". These are red elongate areas on any part of her body that is being stretched. They are unsightly. After the baby, they do not go away, but they change in color to become silvery and somewhat less obvious. But, nonetheless nobody is happy with them. Not all women get stretch marks. It has to do with the type of connective tissue that she was born with. This is similar to varicose veins, which some women get, and others do not. The veins in the legs get large and very prominent. This can be nothing more than an ugly sight or they can develop clots and this then is dangerous. They recede after the baby but they never really go away.

As you can see, by the time she gets to term, she

is not too happy with how she feels or how she looks. You can't help how she looks, but you can help how she feels by telling her you love her.

No matter how prepared she may be, all women approach labor with trepidation. She has heard all the "War Stories" from her friends who like to exaggerate what they went through. Humans live on bad news and avoid telling the good news. We complain about our mates and miss the opportunity to praise them. You too will probably approach labor with some fears. This is normal. It will help if you discuss this with each other. Tell her your fears. You are no less a man because you have concerns. For, after all, she is your wife and the baby is your child. Just tell her you will be there for her.

During labor she will be pricked and prodded. It is fortunate that the routine of giving a woman in labor an enema is no longer in vogue. Blood will be taken and IVs will be started. She will have multiple vaginal examinations that are far from comfortable unless she has had some form of anesthesia. No matter which way the baby comes into the world, she will be cut. If the baby delivers vaginally, she will probably have an episiotomy. That is a cut between the vagina and the anus in order to give more room for the birth of the baby. This cut has short-term effects and some long-term effects. The short-term effects are pain during the post-partum period. This can last for days and up to weeks depending upon the size of the cut, the exact placement of the cut, and the healing process. By the way, during these weeks she may begin to look alluring to you. Wait, the first intercourse after the birth of the baby can be very painful and you need to be patient and gentle. Consider how your privates would feel if you had a large incision made in them.

If the baby delivers by cesarean the abdomen is cut. This takes weeks to heal and is painful. Add to all this the fact that after the baby is born the body produces a great deal of hormones to stimulate the breasts to produce milk. Even if Mom is not going to breast feed, she is going to produce milk. The breasts can become very engorged and painful. This can go on for days.

Post-partum is another bag of worms. This is a time of risk for post-partum depression, a condition over which Mom has no control and can be very dangerous. If you notice any change in your mate's behavior, moods, or outlook on life in general, it would be wise to notify your doctor. Post-partum depression is very treatable if caught in time. It is not a black mark against you or your mate. Take care of it and all will be well.

In this day in age, few households can exist without both parents working. This is very hard on the woman. Emotionally, she does not want to leave the baby, but she knows she must. On the other hand, if she is able to stay home she may be giving up her career. Women today put as much effort into their careers as do men and no man wants to give that up. Women are torn and they need a great deal of help and understanding from you at this time in particular.

I'm telling you this not to make childbirth sound

like a nightmare, but to encourage you to understand what your mate is up against and for you to give her all the love and support that you can muster.

PART TWO

DELIVERY

Chapter Seven

_____

WHERE TO DELIVER AND BY WHOM?

This may seem like a foolish question to those of you who have chosen to have your baby delivered in a hospital by an Obstetrician. But, there are many who feel that they are better off in a Birthing Center or worse – at home.

Many feel that this is quite adequate. Let me say at the onset that they are foolishly playing with their lives and those of their unborn babies.

Allow me to prove my point. An Obstetrician's basic training consists of four years in college, four years in medical school, and four to five years post graduate training specializing in Obstetrics and Gynecology. He may then call himself a specialist.

It does not stop there either. If he wished to be Board Certified he must then pass a very extensive written exam and a year or so later pass an oral exam. If he passes both of these exams he is then "Board Certified" in Obstetrics and Gynecology.

Next, to have a baby anywhere but in a hospital is not smart, certainly, not in the United States of America. All the nonsense about the warmth of a Birthing Center goes out the window when a life-threatening situation occurs. Anyone who tells you that he or she can predict such an occurrence and can cope with that kind of danger outside a hospital is either very ignorant or lying.

Some of the greatest dangers in childbirth come without warning. It is then too late to wish you were in a hospital. All of the so-called hominess of a non-hospital is for naught when you watch your mate slip into a situation that may affect her life and that of your child.

I cannot understand why anyone would want second best for himself or a loved one. When your baby is born in a hospital, all the equipment needed to sustain life is available. There is no need to make hasty arrangements to transfer the mother and your unborn child to a hospital. There is no valuable time lost. I would also recommend if you have more than one hospital to choose from that you choose the hospital with the higher level of care. Tertiary care Obstetrical units give full obstetrical and newborn care. Other hospitals send their problem cases to these facilities. I know you want the best and deserve it. But, any hospital is better than a birthing center or home deliveries. HOME DELIVERIES ARE FOR PIZZA.

Chapter Eight

THE LAST FEW WEEKS

It's possible that sometime in the last few weeks of pregnancy your wife may inform you "she lost her plug". Do not drop everything and start to look for it.

The mouth or opening of the womb contains a gelatinous like substance that acts somewhat like a barrier to keep bacteria from entering the womb and possibly causing an infection. During the last weeks of pregnancy, as the mouth of the womb begins to soften up and shorten the mucous "plug" can become loosened and fall out; as "I LOST MY PLUG". It is not necessarily an indication of anything more than that. All or part of the gelatinous substance came out. She may or may not be going into labor. Should this have happened much earlier in the pregnancy it might have been an indication of an "Incompetent Cervix" where the mouth of the womb could not stay closed throughout the last stages of pregnancy. That situation requires immediate attention. What is sometimes confusing is the differentiation between the lost plug and the rupture of the bag of waters where the baby swims. The plug is gelatinous much like the uncooked egg white. The water that surrounds the baby is normally clear liquid, not viscous and it runs like water. When in doubt, call the doctor.

Chapter Nine

LABOR

Ideally labor would start at the end of pregnancy. If not at the due date, close to it. Such is not the case. Only five percent of all pregnancies deliver on the due date. Anything from two weeks before to two weeks after the due date is considered normal. Should the mother start labor between 20 plus weeks and 37 weeks she will be given drugs to stop labor and steroids to hasten the maturity of the baby's lungs. The hardest part of caring for the premature infant is the immaturity of its lungs and the difficulty in getting oxygen to its organs. Feeding is a small part of the problem. Should labor-stopping drugs work, they will be continued until

37 weeks and stopped. By that time, the baby is out of the woods.

Post maturity is another problem. Not nearly as dangerous as Prematurity but it does have its special challenges. Of course, to the mother one minute after midnight on her due date is post maturity. To the doctor, this is not yet a problem. Anywhere from one to two weeks past the due date is to be dealt with.

How is Post Maturity dealt with? First off a BPP (Biophysical Profile) can be done. This is an examination with ultrasound of the baby. It uses markers to evaluate the fetal status. They are: the amount of fluid surrounding the baby, fetal movement, fetal tone (movement of finger and toes) and fetal breathing. The baby is given two points for each good marker. Eight points is fine, six is questionable and anything less requires immediate attention.

The present day method of induction for Post Mature infants is to insert a special suppository in the vagina whose function is to soften and open up the mouth of the womb. Mostly, this is done over night in the hospital. The suppository is then removed and Pitocin is started in a very dilute solution, intravenously. An automatic pump is then used to slowly administer small doses and to increase this by small increments until labor is achieved.

A word about Pitocin. To the average patient this has become a scary substance. They have been told that it causes labor pains. That is true. But, labor that starts by itself also causes pain. The only difference between the pains is that one is started by pitocin and one is started by spontaneous labor. What the doctor is trying to do in using pitocin is to mimic labor. That's induced labor. It is no different than the real thing. Labor pains hurt.

Now, let's talk about the real thing. Nature has many different ways of ushering in labor. All are different. But, unfortunately, pain is always there. If it were possible to have labor without any pain most babies would be born at home without warning.

Some of the early signs of labor are: lower back pain, vaginal bleeding, leaking or rupturing of the bag of water, uterine contractions that occur every five minutes or less and increasing in intensity (becoming more painful).

Let's discuss these uterine contractions. The uterus is an organ in the female body whose sole function is to be the house for the unborn baby. There is a cavity inside the uterus that builds a lining each month to receive a conceptus (fetus). If no pregnancy occurs the lining is shed and the cycle begins again. Hormones that are secreted into the blood stream at different intervals control this menstrual cycle. As a muscular organ the uterus "delivers" the baby by contracting. A hormone is released into the blood stream, oxytocin, and travels to the uterus causing the muscle fiber to tighten and contract. These contractions eventually cause the opening of the uterus or cervix to dilate and the baby moves from the uterus to the birth canal or vagina and then finally passes into the world.

However, in an attempt to keep the labor and

delivery process a true mystery nature devised something we call Braxton-Hicks contractions or "false" labor pains. The key word to understand Braxton-Hicks contractions is the word "false" meaning they don't cause the delivery of the baby.

About halfway through pregnancy the hormone oxytocin is released into the blood stream causing the muscles of the uterus to contract. Let's say that the uterus now starts training for delivery. Pregnant patients sometime feel these contractions and sometimes they don't. Either way the contractions do happen. They are mild and of short duration. Sometimes they are perceived as baby's movements, bladder spasms, back spasms, etc.

The important thing to remember about "false" labor pains is just that, they do not cause the delivery of the baby. They contract the uterine muscle but this has no effect on the cervix and therefore the baby cannot pass from the uterus to the birth canal. Pregnant women often feel these contractions more as they get closer to their due date. Often these contractions can become regular and form a pattern but their intensity (painfulness) and duration (length of time that they last) never changes. It is therefore important to pay attention to the signals that the body gives.

Many times women mistaken early labor for Braxton-Hicks contractions but when the contractions become more painful and they last longer then, the real labor process has begun. The bottom line is that the only way to identify labor contraction versus false labor contractions is to examine the cervix for changes. This is done by the physician. Sometimes women will "think" that they are in labor and they call the doctor or go to the labor room only to find out that the cervix has not changed and therefore labor has not yet begun. Sometimes hydration (giving water by mouth or I.V.) will stop these false labor pains. Nothing is lost for eventually she will go into labor.

The Stages of Labor. For the sake of description labor is divided into three stages. The first stage is from the start of labor till full dilation. The second stage is from full dilation till delivery of the baby and the third stage is the delivery of the placenta (also called the afterbirth).

This requires more explanation. First off imagine the uterus or womb as a big hollow muscle with a long thick neck at one end. The baby is inside the hollow muscle and the neck (cervix) sits into the top of the vagina. The canal or cervix is about two inches long and it keeps the baby from leaving the hollow muscle. When labor starts this hollow muscle starts contracting (squeezing), which in turn makes the long closed cervix start to shorten and open. With each contraction (labor pain) the cervix gets shorter and opens. This shortening is called effacement. Fifty percent effacement means just that, it is fifty percent shortened. When it is 100 percent effaced it is a thin as a football's pigskin. The opening of the cervix goes from a fingertip to ten centimeters, which is called full dilatation. This is the end of the first stage. From there on the baby descend through the vagina (or birth canal) till it is born. If you hear someone in the labor room mention plus one or plus two, or minus one, etc. they are telling whoever is listening as to where a certain point on the fetal head is in relationship to a point in the mother's pelvis. Minuses are high and pluses are low. Plus three is really getting there.

After the birth of the baby, the hollow muscle (uterus) squeezes down as tight as it can and in doing so it shears off the placenta (afterbirth) into the vagina and from there it is delivered by the doctor. Usually the cord, which connects the baby to the afterbirth, is cut by this third stage and the doctor then gives his attention to any repair work that needs to be done. Be it an episiotomy or any spontaneous lacerations.

Before we go any further it would be nice to talk about the mother's need for reduction of the pain. Labor is pain, but that doesn't mean that Mom has to grin and bear it. This is not the 20th century but the 21st century and great strides have been made in anesthesia. The greatest stride, as far as labor is concerned, is what I would like to call the "**BIG E**" or Epidural. This is a regional type of anesthesia, which allows the mother to be wide-awake through out labor and delivery and feel no pain. It makes no difference what type of delivery, be spontaneous, forceps or even Cesarean Section a good epidural is a Godsend. How is it done? An anesthesiologist places a needle between two spinal vertebrae in the lower back and then threads a thin plastic tube through the needle into the space inside the vertebrae, removes the needle and administers the anesthetic agent through this tube on a continuous basis, either by pump or by patient controlled injection or both; thereby keeping the patient comfortable through out the whole process of labor and delivery.

The Induction of Labor. After having discussed Labor, we need to explain the Induction of Labor. The term itself is self-explanatory. It means to artificially start labor rather than to await the spontaneous (natural) onset of labor.

There are many reasons why one would want to start labor before it begins on its own. One of them, that most would understand and agree with, is in the situation of a woman who already has given birth to a previous child but whose labor was too rapid for here to make it to the hospital. Most would want to induce her next baby before labor begins on its own and thereby deliver in the hospital.

Another situation is what is called a post dates pregnancy. This is when the pregnancy goes past its due date. One of the debated points is when is it post dates. Patients believe it is the next day after the due date. Physicians seem to have different ideas. Anywhere from one to two weeks past term. The reasons are that it is generally agreed that nothing good happens past the due date and there is the fear that the placenta, that nourishes and gives oxygen to the baby, may have gone beyond its maturity and in its aging it has decreased its ability to do its job.

Diabetes is another situation. Most feel that once a well-controlled diabetic reaches her due date, she and the baby are best served by delivery. Induction is frequently chosen over Cesarean Section. But, at times, the baby of a diabetic may be too big for a vaginal delivery and Cesarean is performed.

Pregnancy induced hypertension and its related situations are frequently an indication for induction.

The list goes on and on. In a word, inductions are done either for the mother's well being or the baby's. And usually it is best for both of them.

Induction of labor. There are many ways of inducing labor. Most of the variables have to do with the situation of the cervix (mouth of the womb). If it is soft, thinned out and somewhat opened one can go directly to induction. If it is not so, then there are ways to prime the cervix and get it ready for induction.

Some of the so called ripening or priming methods are: The placement of a catheter through the mouth of the womb and inflating a rubber bulb at the end of the catheter and thereby stretching the cervical opening. One can also use a laminaria, which is a dried out and very compact strip of Japanese seaweed. This is about the size of a soda straw. It is left in over night and as it rehydrates itself with liquid it swells up and opens the cervix. A third method uses a suppository that contains prostaglandin (a hormone that acts upon the uterus to ripen up and open up the cervix.) This also is left in for up to twelve hours.

Once the cervix is ripened up, either by itself or through one of the above methods, induction is begun. The usual method is to give a weak solution of pitocin through an I.V. This is started at a very low dosage and is progressively increased until labor has begun. At that time, once labor has started, the pitocin can be discontinued and labor will still go on. If it doesn't it can always be restarted.

During the induction the fetal heart is monitored. This can be done either electronically or by sound. In the case of sound a microphone like transducer is placed on the mother's abdomen. The electronic surveillance requires that the bag of waters is ruptured and a scalp electrode is placed on the fetal scalp. This is a far more accurate method in that it is a direct method and does not immobilize the mother as much as the transducer does but it does require that the bag of waters be broken. That in itself can also be a good surveillance of fetal well being in that the quality of the fluid gives very good evidence of how the baby is doing. For that reason, most physicians will rupture the bag of water once it can be done safely.

Types of Deliveries: Actually, there are only two types of deliveries: vaginal and abdominal. But, there are many variables to each of these.

As far as the vaginal deliveries are concerned, the first variety is called a spontaneous vaginal delivery. The "spontaneous" part has nothing to do with an "out of the blue" situation. What it really means is a delivery in which the mother simply pushes the baby out into the hands of the catcher, be it a doctor, a nurse, or even a taxi cab driver.

The second variety is when the doctor helps the mother in her efforts to deliver. He is helping her by using various instruments that allow him to pull the baby out. The pull can be done by using a vacuum cup that attaches to the infant's scalp. This can also be done by the use of forceps that are cupped next to the infant's cheeks. Here there is a great debate in medicine concerning whether or not these are valuable and safe instruments. I will only state that like any instrument they are only as good as the person who uses them. Experience and gentleness and knowing when to use them, how to use them, and when to call it quits is probably the best judge. Knowing how to use them can avoid Cesarean Sections. Talk to your doctor about this.

The third type of vaginal delivery is a breech delivery. This is when the baby is trying to exit its mother and enter the world "butt" first. Up until recently, most breech deliveries were vaginal, provided they fit. Now, somewhat due to lack of training and experience most breech babies are delivered by Cesarean Section. Where this becomes a problem is when there are twins and the first one is coming headfirst and the second one is coming as a breech. Do you deliver the head first one vaginally and then deliver the breech by Cesarean Section? My feelings are that if you are not capable of delivering a breech vaginally then you might as well deliver them both by Cesarean Section.

Other vaginal delivery problems arise when the baby may be coming headfirst but the head is either turned the wrong way or the head is tilted. To explain this you need to realize that the best position for a baby to be in for a vaginal delivery is when he or she is facing the floor and leading with the back of the head. This presents the smallest diameters to the mother's pelvis. If the baby is facing the ceiling, this is no good. What is even worse is when the baby is coming face first. If, in the face-first, the chin is down and forehead is up, it's possible. If it is chin up and forehead down, it's possible but difficult. Most of these abnormal head presentations require either a change or a Cesarean.

Abdominal (Cesarean Section) delivery. The cesarean is accomplished by either putting Mom to sleep or giving a regional block via her spine. The incision, year's ago, was from the naval to below the hairline. Most present day abdominal incisions are the so-called "bikini" incision; they follow a line just below where a bikini would be. The incision in the uterus also varies. Up and down or sideways. Side ways is the best in that it cuts into an area that does not bleed as much as a cut that goes up the front of the uterus. It also is in an area that does not have as great a risk of rupture in a subsequent pregnancy as does an up and down one.

Episiotomy. An Episiotomy is a cut that is made from the back of the entrance of the vagina. It can be made straight back toward the rectum or to the left or right at an angle to the side. Its rational is to make the opening of the vagina bigger and thereby aide in the delivery of the baby. If you consider that the entrance to the vagina has a diameter of about one to two inches and the diameter of the baby's head is close to twice that. Considering that, then either an episiotomy is done or the opening is stretched or the opening rips enough to accommodate the birth.

Up until about five to ten years ago, episiotomies were routine. It was believed to be the best method to preserve the mother's vagina. Recently, there is much debate concerning this. It would take too many pages to explain it all. Therefore, I will give you my opinion. After delivering close to 10,000 babies, I am convinced that if the baby is to deliver vaginally, it is better to increase the diameter of the vagina by doing an episiotomy and then sew up a nice clean incision than to stretch or have to rip and leave a ragged wound to be repaired.

Newborn circumcision. I do approve of circumcision of the newborn male. With that said, I must admit that besides ritual circumcision for Jewish males there is little if any medical reason to have one done. I imagine that most circumcised fathers probably would want there sons to be circumcised. There is also the fear that if the baby is not circumcised he might be made fun of by a circumcised male when he grows up, considering that most male babies today are circumcised. But, there are many new ethnic groups that are now living in America who do not circumcise their male babies. Female circumcision is another thing. That is shear mutilation of the female baby and aught never to be done.

There is also a trend to use some form of anesthesia for newborn circumcision. This is either done with an anesthetic cream (that doesn't really work) rubbed on the penis around the foreskin that is to be removed. There is also an injection that can be used by injecting an anesthetic agent around the foreskin. My impression is this. I have never known an adult man who remembers his circumcision. I can't believe that it causes any psychological harm. There is no evidence for that. Circumcised Americans and Jews around the globe have no more hang ups than the rest of the uncircumcised world.

As far as the baby's reaction to being circumcised, they all react the same with or without anesthesia. They are first strapped down to a plastic board; their arms are strapped down, as are their legs. This is when they all protest by crying and continue to do so until they are released from the bondage. Anesthetized or not they all cry. Stick them with a needle or massage them with cream, they all protest. Prior to cutting off the foreskin, without anesthesia, the skin is squeezed in a clamp, which deadens the area, which is then cut. There is no increase in fetal protestation at that point of cutting. After that it's all over. The baby is then released and stops crying and is looking for Mom and food.

PART THREE

POSTPARTUM

Chapter Ten

POSTPARTUM

Barring a complication, once the baby is born and the placenta (afterbirth) is out, labor is all over. Now begins the postpartum phase. If an episiotomy was done it is now repaired. If birth was by cesarean, the uterus and abdominal incision is closed. Once the mother is stable, she is transferred to her bed on the postpartum unit and the baby goes to the nursery for preliminary observation. Over the next few days the mother will have what is called lochia. This is vaginal discharge that goes from outright red blood to brown to beige to clear to nothing. This can take weeks. Usually all bleeding and discharge is gone by six weeks when she comes into the doctor's office for her postpartum check up.

As I have explained, the uterus is a hollow organ that is made up of a muscular wall. This muscle needs to contract in order to expel the baby but what is important is how it sees to it that the mother does not bleed to death after the birth. Let me explain. The uterus has a large blood supply during pregnancy in order to supply the fetus with nourishment and oxygen for its growth. These vessels are interlaced through the muscle fiber of the uterus. Once the baby is born the muscle contracts and squeezes these vessels down and thereby control the bleeding. It is for this reason that after the birth of the baby, the mother is given pitocin in order to keep the uterus contracted and thereby control the bleeding. The mother's body takes over and controls the bleeding. If she doesn't, she can be given other agents, either by injection or by mouth. Postpartum hemorrhage can be very dangerous. It can lead to the need to remove the uterus in order to save the mother. It is for this reason that the nurses keep sharp vigilance on the postpartum uterine contractions and the amount of vaginal bleeding.

Breast-feeding. I would highly recommend that the mother breast-feed. First, and not necessarily the most important reason is that breast-feeding makes the uterus contract and lessen the postpartum bleeding in amount and duration. Breast-feeding mothers get to the point of no more bleeding and discharge sooner than do non breast-feeding Moms. From the baby's point of view breast-feeding gives them antibodies to combat many childhood illnesses along with the best nourishment possible. Formulas can't compete. This is not meant to make non-breast feeding mothers feel guilty. There are reasons not to breast-feed. Some mother's don't make sufficient milk to adequately nourish the baby. Some mothers work. Some mothers have an adversity to breast feeding and should be respected. It's not as if there was no alternative. We do have other means of feeding the baby. If it works and it is good for both the mother and the baby, go for it. If not, let it be. This should not be the father's choice. It must be the mother's.

Most mothers have postpartum "blues". It is just that. It's a little let down after some very hard work. Just support her and let her know that you are there for her and you love her. It is short lived. But, stay alert to it. If, per chance, it seems like it's getting worse and she is getting depressed, call the doctor. True postpartum depression is very dangerous but very treatable if caught in time. Mom has NO control over this. Don't just expect her to duke-it-out. She NEEDS HELP. Keep the so-called well-meaning mothers, mother-in-laws and friends away. They all seem to think that they know the answer to every problem. They don't. Call the doctor.

Sex. Sexual intercourse is out until the postpartum check up. It is important for the doctor to check Mom and to advise her of when it is safe to resume. Respect this. It is also important to discuss methods of family planning with the doctor before you accidentally start an unwanted pregnancy. Don't rely on breast-feeding as birth control. Granted ovulation and breast-feeding usually don't go hand in hand but women can become pregnant while breast-feeding. Therefore, breast feed for the baby but not for family planning.

Birth control methods can be divided into temporary and permanent. The temporary can be divided into barrier methods and medical methods and so called natural family planning methods. Barriers are condoms used by the male or diaphragms used by the female or the not too popular IUDs. The condoms and diaphragms both stand in the way of sperm and eggs meeting. The IUDs are placed inside the uterus and it is believed that they too interfere with egg and sperm union. Some think that the IUDs interfere with implantation of the fertilized egg (possibly abortifacients).

The medical methods are birth control pills taken by mouth, birth control patches applied to the skin, injection of hormones or implantation of hormone pellets placed under the skin (not too popular).

Natural Family Planning methods are without pills or barriers. The thought is that by using female temperature changes and certain changes in the viscosity of the cervical mucous that fertile days and unfertile days can be predicted and thereby the ability to know when to and when not to have intercourse. Many people who are breast-feeding think that they can combine breast-feeding and natural family planning to be more successful in avoiding a pregnancy. Such is not the case. The physiology of the female who is breast-feeding and that of the non-breast feeding female is totally different. The temperature shifts and mucous changes do not exist in the breast-feeding female.

Permanent Methods are male sterilization and female sterilization. The female is done in the hospital under anesthesia. Both Fallopian Tubes are either tied, clamped or cauterized. It can be done through the belly button using a telescope or through a small incision in the lower abdomen.

Male sterilization is usually done in the doctor's office with local anesthesia. A small incision is made in both sides of the scrotum (sack that hold the testicles) and the ducts that transports the sperm out of the testicles is tied and cut. The incision is closed and the man can go home. One of the big differences between male and female sterilization is that the female is rendered sterile right away but the male is not. He needs to clear out sperm that is on the other side of the cut. This can take up to ten ejaculations. A semen analysis should be done to verify that there are no more sperm.

A closing word about sex. The first intercourse after a baby, especially after a vaginal birth with repairs of lacerations or episiotomy, can be painful for the female. Please, be gentle and use a lot of K-Y Jelly. In time it will work out but don't expect your wife to be free of discomfort.

Well, you've made it to the end. I want to thank you for taking the time to read this. I do so hope that it will be of some help to you as you approach fatherhood. But, please remember that even though fatherhood starts with the birth of the child, it does not end there. It goes on and on and it can be not only your greatest challenge but more important your greatest reward.

ISBN 141203644-5